The Definitive Diabetic Diet Cooking Guide for Beginners

Get Back in Shape and Manage Your Weight with Amazingly Healthy Desserts

Danielle Woods

contained within this document, including, but not limited to, — errors, omissions, or inaccuracies.

Table of contents

Hot Kamut With Peaches, Walnuts, And Coconut

Preparation Time : 10 minutes

Cooking Time : 35 minutes

Servings : 04

Ingredients :

- Toasted coconut, 4 tbsp.
- Toasted and chopped walnuts, .5 c
- Chopped dried peaches, 8
- Coconut milk, 3 c
- Kamut cereal, 1 c

Directions :

1. Mix the coconut milk into a saucepan and allow it to warm up. When it begins simmering, add in the Kamut. Let this cook about 15 minutes, while stirring every now and then.

2. When done, divide evenly into bowls and top with the toasted coconut, walnuts, and peaches.

3. You could even go one more and add some fresh berries.

Nutrition : Calories: 156; Protein: 5.8 g; Carbohydrates: 25 g; Fiber: 6 g

Overnight "Oats"

Preparation Time : 5 minutes

Cooking Time : 0 minutes

Servings : 04

Ingredients :

- Berry of choice, .5 c
- Walnut butter, .5 tbsp.
- Burro banana, .5
- Ginger, .5 tsp.
- Coconut milk, .5 c
- Hemp seeds, .5 c

Directions:

1. Put the hemp seeds, salt, and coconut milk into a glass jar. Mix well.

2. Place the lid on the jar then put in the refrigerator to sit overnight.

3. The next morning, add the ginger, berries, and banana. Stir well and enjoy.

Nutrition : Calories: 139; Fat: 4.1 g; Protein: 9 g; Sugar: 7 g

Blueberry Cupcakes

Preparation Time : 15 minutes

Cooking Time : 40 minutes

Servings : 04

Ingredients :

- Grapeseed oil
- Sea salt, .5 tsp.
- Sea moss gel, .25 c
- Agave, .3 c
- Blueberries, .5 c
- Teff flour, .75 c
- Spelt flour, .75 c
- Coconut milk, 1 c

Directions :

1. Warm your oven to 365. Place paper liners into a muffin tin.
2. Place sea moss gel, sea salt, agave, flour, and milk in large bowl. Mix well to combine. Gently fold in blueberries.
3. Gently pour batter into paper liners. Place in oven and bake 30 minutes.
4. They are done if they have turned a nice golden color, and they spring back when you touch them.

Nutrition : Calories: 85; Fat: 0.7 g; Carbohydrates: 12 g; Protein: 1.4 g; Fiber: 5 g

Brazil Nut Cheese

Preparation Time : 2 hours

Cooking Time : 0 minutes

Servings : 4

Ingredients :

- Grapeseed oil, 2 tsp.

- Water, 1.5 c

- Hemp milk, 1.5 c

- Cayenne, .5 tsp.

- Onion powder, 1 tsp.

- Juice of .5 lime

- Sea salt, 2 tsp.

- Brazil nuts, 1 lb.

- Onion powder, 1 tsp.

Directions :

1. You will need to start process by soaking the Brazil nuts in some water. You just put the nuts into a bowl and make sure the water covers them. Soak no less than two hours or overnight. Overnight would be best.

2. Now you need to put everything except water into a food processor or blender.

3. Add just .5 cups water and blend for two minutes

4. Continue adding .5 cup water and blending until you have the consistency you want.

5. Scrape into an airtight container and enjoy.

Nutrition : Calories: 187; Protein: 4.1 g; Fat: 19 g; Carbs: 3.3 g; Fiber: 2.1 g

Slow Cooker Peaches

Preparation Time : 10 minutes

Cooking Time : 4 hours 20 minutes

Servings : 4-6

Ingredients:

- 4 cups peaches, sliced
- 2/3 cup rolled oats
- 1/3 cup Bisques
- 1/4 teaspoon cinnamon
- 1/2 cup brown sugar
- 1/2 cup granulated sugar

Directions :

1. Spray the slow cooker pot with a cooking spray.
2. Mix oats, Bisques, cinnamon and all the sugars in the pot.
3. Add peaches and stir well to combine. Cook on low for 4-6 hours.

Nutrition : 617 Calories; 3.6 g Fat; 13 g Total Carbs; 9 g Protein

Pumpkin Custard

Preparation Time : 10 minutes

Cooking Time : 2 hours 30 minutes

Servings : 6

Ingredients:

- 1/2 cup almond flour
- 4 eggs
- 1 cup pumpkin puree
- 1/2 cup stevia/erythritol blend , granulated
- 1/8 teaspoon sea salt
- 1 teaspoon vanilla extract or maple flavoring
- 4 tablespoons butter, ghee, or coconut oil melted
- 1 teaspoon pumpkin pie spice

Directions :

1. Grease or spray a slow cooker with butter or coconut oil spray.

2. In a medium mixing bowl, beat the eggs until smooth. Then add in the sweetener.

3. To the egg mixture, add in the pumpkin puree along with vanilla or maple extract.

4. Then add almond flour to the mixture along with the pumpkin pie spice and salt. Add melted butter, coconut oil or ghee.

5. Transfer the mixture into a slow cooker. Close the lid. Cook for 2-2 ¾ hours on low.

6. When through, serve with whipped cream, and then sprinkle with little nutmeg if need be. Enjoy!

7. Set slow-cooker to the low setting. Cook for 2-2.45 hours, and begin checking at the two-hour mark. Serve warm with stevia sweetened whipped cream and a sprinkle of nutmeg.

Nutrition : 147 Calories; 12 g Fat; 4 g Total Carbs; 5 g Protein

Blueberry Lemon Custard Cake

Preparation Time : 10 minutes

Cooking Time : 3 hours

Servings : 12

Ingredients:

- 6 eggs, separated
- 2 cups light cream
- 1/2 cup coconut flour
- 1/2 teaspoon salt
- 2 teaspoon lemon zest
- 1/2 cup granulated sugar substitute
- 1/3 cup lemon juice
- 1/2 cup blueberries fresh
- 1 teaspoon lemon liquid stevia

Directions :

1. Into a stand mixer, add the egg whites and whip them well until stiff peaks have formed; set aside.

2. Whisk the yolks together with the remaining ingredients except blueberries, to form batter.

3. When done, fold egg whites into the formed batter a little at a time until slightly combined.

4. Grease the crock pot and then pour in the mixture. Then sprinkle batter with the blueberries.

5. Close the lid then cook for 3 hours on low. When the cooking time is over, open the lid and let cool for an

hour, and then let chill in the refrigerator for at least 2 hours or overnight.

6. Serve cold with little sugar free whipped cream and enjoy!

Nutrition : 165 Calories; 10 g Fat; 14 g Total Carbs; 4 g Protein

Sugar Free Carrot Cake

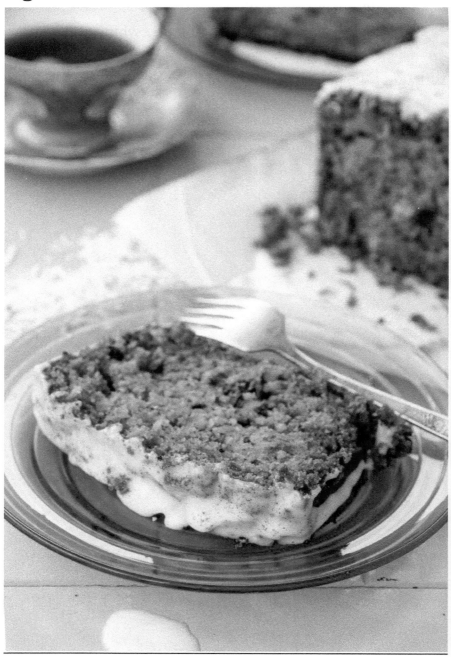

Cooking Time : 4 hours

Servings : 8

Ingredients :

For Carrot cake:

- 2 eggs
- 1 1/2 almond flour
- 1/2 cup butter, melted
- ¼ cup heavy cream
- 1 teaspoon baking powder
- 1 teaspoon vanilla extract or almond extract, optional
- 1 cup sugar substitute
- 1 cup carrots, finely shredded
- 1 teaspoon cinnamon
- ¼ teaspoon nutmeg
- 1/8 teaspoon allspice
- 1 teaspoon ginger
- 1/2 teaspoon baking soda

For cream cheese frosting:

- 1 cup confectioner's sugar substitute
- ¼ cup butter, softened
- 1 teaspoon almond extract
- 4 oz. cream cheese, softened

Directions :

1. Grease a loaf pan well and then set it aside.

2. Using a mixer, combine butter together with eggs, vanilla, sugar substitute and heavy cream in a mixing bowl, until well blended.

3. Combine almond flour together with baking powder, spices and the baking soda in another bowl until well blended.

4. When done, combine the wet ingredients together with the dry ingredients until well blended, and then stir in carrots.

5. Pour the mixer into the prepared loaf pan, and then place the pan into a slow cooker on a trivet. Add 1 cup water inside.

6. Cook for about 4-5 hours on low. Be aware that the cake will be very moist.

7. When the cooking time is over, let the cake cool completely.

8. To prepare the cream cheese frosting: blend the cream cheese together with extract, butter and powdered sugar substitute until frosting is formed.

9. Top the cake with the frosting.

Nutrition : 299 Calories; 25.4 g Fat; 15 g Total Carbs; 4 g Protein

Sugar Free Chocolate Molten Lava Cake

Preparation Time : 10 minutes

Cooking Time : 3 hours

Servings : 12

Ingredients:

- 3 egg yolks
- 1 1/2 cups Swerve sweetener , divided
- 1 teaspoon baking powder
- 1/2 cup flour, gluten free
- 3 whole eggs
- 5 tablespoons cocoa powder , unsweetened, divided
- 4 oz. chocolate chips , sugar free
- 1/2 teaspoon salt
- 1/2 teaspoon vanilla liquid stevia
- 1/2 cup butter, melted, cooled
- 2 cups hot water
- 1 teaspoon vanilla extract

Directions :

1. Grease the crockpot well with cooking spray.

2. Whisk 1 ¼ cups of swerve together with flour, salt, baking powder and 3 tablespoons cocoa powder in a bowl.

3. Stir the cooled melted butter together with eggs, yolks, liquid stevia and the vanilla extract in a separate bowl.

4. When done, add the wet ingredients to the dry ingredient until nicely combined, and then pour the mixture into the prepared crock pot.

5. Then top the mixture in the crockpot with chocolate chips.

6. Whisk the rest of the swerve sweetener and the remaining cocoa powder with the hot water, and then pour this mixture over the chocolate chips top.

7. Close the lid and cook for 3 hours on low. When the cooking time is over, let cool a bit and then serve. Enjoy!

Nutrition : 157 Calories; 13 g Fat; 10.5 g Total Carbs; 3.9 g Protein

Chocolate Quinoa Brownies

Preparation Time : 10 minutes

Cooking Time : 2 hours

Servings : 16

Ingredients :

- 2 eggs
- 3 cups quinoa, cooked
- 1 teaspoon vanilla liquid stevia
- 1 ¼ chocolate chips, sugar free
- 1 teaspoon vanilla extract
- 1/3 cup flaxseed ground
- ¼ teaspoon salt
- 1/3 cup cocoa powder, unsweetened
- 1/2 teaspoon baking powder
- 1 teaspoon pure stevia extract
- 1/2 cup applesauce, unsweetened

Sugar- frees frosting:

- ¼ cup heavy cream
- 1 teaspoon chocolate liquid stevia
- ¼ cup cocoa powder, unsweetened
- 1/2 teaspoon vanilla extract

Directions:

1. Add all the ingredients to a food processor. Then process until well incorporated.

23

2. Line a crock pot with a parchment paper, and then spread the batter into the lined pot.

3. Close the lid and cook for 4 hours on LOW or 2 hours on HIGH. Let cool.

4. Prepare the frosting. Whisk all the ingredients together and then microwave for 20 seconds. Taste and adjust on sweetener if desired.

5. When the frosting is ready, stir it well again and then pour it over the sliced brownies.

6. Serve and enjoy!

Nutrition : 133 Calories; 7.9 g Fat; 18.4 g Total Carbs; 4.3 g Protein

Blueberry Crisp

Preparation Time : 10 minutes

Cooking Time : 3-4 hours

Servings : 10

Ingredients:

- 1/4 cup butter, melted
- 24 oz. blueberries, frozen
- 3/4 teaspoon salt
- 1 1/2 cups rolled oats, coarsely ground
- 3/4 cup almond flour, blanched
- 1/4 cup coconut oil, melted
- 6 tablespoons sweetener
- 1 cup pecans or walnuts, coarsely chopped

Directions :

1. Using a non-stick cooking spray, spray the slow cooker pot well.

2. Into a bowl, add ground oats and chopped nuts along with salt, blanched almond flour, brown sugar, stevia granulated sweetener, and then stir in the coconut/butter mixture. Stir well to combine.

3. When done, spread crisp topping over blueberries. Cook for 3-4 hours, until the mixture has become bubbling hot and you can smell the blueberries.

4. Serve while still hot with the whipped cream or the ice cream if desired. Enjoy!

Nutrition : 261 Calories; 16.6 g Fat; 32 g Total Carbs; 4 g Protein

Maple Custard

Preparation Time : 10 minutes

Cooking Time : 2 hours

Servings : 6

Ingredients:

- 1 teaspoon maple extract
- 2 egg yolks
- 1 cup heavy cream
- 2 eggs
- 1/2 cup whole milk
- 1/4 teaspoon salt
- 1/4 cup Sukrin Gold or any sugar-free brown sugar substitute
- 1/2 teaspoon cinnamon

Directions :

1. Combine all ingredients together in a blender, process well.

2. Grease 6 ramekins and then pour the batter evenly into each ramekin.

3. To the bottom of the slow cooker, add 4 ramekins and then arrange the remaining 2 against the side of a slow cooker, and not at the top of bottom ramekins.

4. Close the lid and cook on high for 2 hours, until the center is cooked through but the middle is still jiggly.

5. Let cool at a room temperature for an hour after removing from the slow cooker, and then chill in the fridge for at least 2 hours.

6. Serve and enjoy with a sprinkle of cinnamon and little sugar free whipped cream.

Nutrition : 190 Calories; 18 g Fat; 2 g Total Carbs; 4 g Protein

Raspberry Cream Cheese Coffee Cake

Preparation Time : 10 minutes

Cooking Time : 4 hours

Servings : 12

Ingredients:

- 1 1/4 almond flour
- 2/3 cup water
- 1/2 cup Swerve
- 3 eggs
- 1/4 cup coconut flour
- 1/4 cup protein powder
- 1/4 teaspoon salt
- 1/2 teaspoon vanilla extract
- 1 1/2 teaspoon baking powder
- 6 tablespoons butter, melted

For the Filling:

- 1 1/2 cup fresh raspberries
- 8 oz. cream cheese
- 1 large egg
- 1/3 cup powdered Swerve
- 2 tablespoon whipping cream

Directions :

1. Grease the slow cooker pot. Prepare the cake batter. In a bowl, combine almond flour together with coconut

flour, sweetener, baking powder, protein powder and salt, and then stir in the melted butter along with eggs and water until well combined. Set aside.

2. Prepare the filling. Beat cream cheese thoroughly with the sweetener until have smoothened, and then beat in whipping cream along with the egg and vanilla extract until well combined.

3. Assemble the cake. Spread around 2/3 of batter in the slow cooker as you smoothen the top using a spatula or knife.

4. Pour cream cheese mixture over the batter in the pan, evenly spread it, and then sprinkle with raspberries. Add the rest of batter over filling.

5. Cook for 3-4 hours on low. Let cool completely.

6. Serve and enjoy!

Nutrition : 239 Calories; 19.18 g Tat; 6.9 g Total Carbs; 7.5 g Protein

Pumpkin Pie Bars

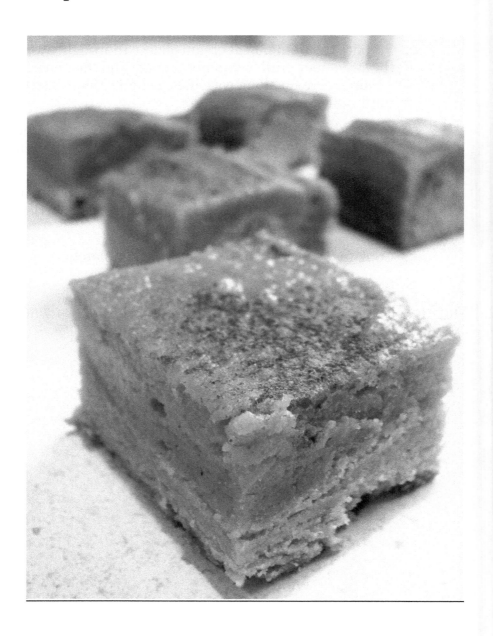

Preparation Time : 10 minutes

Cooking Time : 3 hours

Servings : 16

Ingredients :

For the Crust:

- 3/4 cup coconut, shredded
- 4 tablespoons butter, unsalted, softened
- 1/4 cup cocoa powder, unsweetened
- 1/4 teaspoon salt
- 1/2 cup raw sunflower seeds or sunflower seed flour
- 1/4 cup confectioners Swerve

Filling:

- 2 teaspoons cinnamon liquid stevia
- 1 cup heavy cream
- 1 can pumpkin puree
- 6 eggs
- 1 tablespoon pumpkin pie spice
- 1/2 teaspoon salt
- 1 tablespoon vanilla extract
- 1/2 cup sugar-free chocolate chips, optional

Directions :

1. Add all the crust ingredients to a food processor. Then process until fine crumbs are formed.

2. Grease the slow cooker pan well. When done, press crust mixture onto the greased bottom.

3. In a stand mixer, combine all the ingredients for the filling, and then blend well until combined.

4. Top the filling with chocolate chips if using, and then pour the mixture onto the prepared crust.

5. Close the lid and cook for 3 hours on low. Open the lid and let cool for at least 30 minutes, and then place the slow cooker into the refrigerator for at least 3 hours.

6. Slice the pumpkin pie bar and serve it with sugar free whipped cream. Enjoy!

Nutrition : 169 Calories; 15 g Fat; 6 g Total Carbs; 4 g Protein

Dark Chocolate Cake

Preparation Time : 10 minutes

Cooking Time : 3 hours

Servings : 10

Ingredients:

- 1 cup almond flour
- 3 eggs
- 2 tablespoons almond flour
- 1/4 teaspoon salt
- 1/2 cup Swerve Granular
- 3/4 teaspoon vanilla extract
- 2/3 cup almond milk, unsweetened
- 1/2 cup cocoa powder
- 6 tablespoons butter, melted
- 1 1/2 teaspoon baking powder
- 3 tablespoons unflavored whey protein powder or egg white protein powder
- 1/3 cup sugar-free chocolate chips , optional

Directions :

1. Grease the slow cooker well.

2. Whisk the almond flour together with cocoa powder, sweetener, whey protein powder, salt and baking powder in a bowl. Then stir in butter along with almond milk, eggs and the vanilla extract until well combined, and then stir in the chocolate chips if desired.

3. When done, pour into the slow cooker. Allow to cook for 2-2 1/2 hours on low.

4. When through, turn off the slow cooker and let the cake cool for about 20-30 minutes.

5. When cooled, cut the cake into pieces and serve warm with lightly sweetened whipped cream. Enjoy!

Nutrition : 205 Calories; 17 g Fat; 8.4 g Total Carbs; 12 g Protein

Lemon Custard

Preparation Time : 10 minutes

Cooking Time : 3 hours

Servings : 4

Ingredients :

- 2 cups whipping cream or coconut cream
- 5 egg yolks
- 1 tablespoon lemon zest
- 1 teaspoon vanilla extract
- 1/4 cup fresh lemon juice, squeezed
- 1/2 teaspoon liquid stevia
- Lightly sweetened whipped cream

Directions :

1. Whisk egg yolks together with lemon zest, liquid stevia, lemon zest and vanilla in a bowl, and then whisk in heavy cream.

2. Divide the mixture among 4 small jars or ramekins.

3. To the bottom of a slow cooker add a rack, and then add ramekins on top of the rack and add enough water to cover half of ramekins.

4. Close the lid and cook for 3 hours on low. Remove ramekins.

5. Let cool to room temperature, and then place into the refrigerator to cool completely for about 3 hours.

6. When through, top with the whipped cream and serve. Enjoy!

Nutrition : 319 Calories; 30 g Fat; 3 g Total Carbs; 7 g Protein

Baked Stuffed Pears

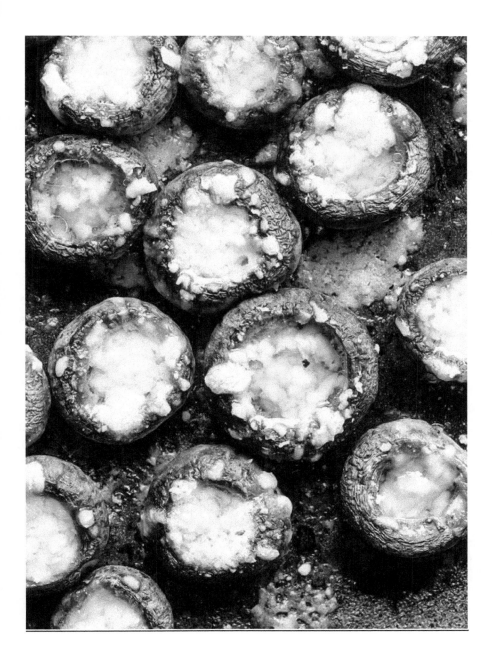

Preparation Time : 15 minutes

Cooking Time : 35 minutes

Servings : 4

Ingredients :

- Agave syrup, 4 tbsp.
- Cloves, .25 tsp.
- Chopped walnuts, 4 tbsp.
- Currants, 1 c
- Pears, 4

Directions :

1. Make sure your oven has been warmed to 375.
2. Slice the pears in two lengthwise and remove the core. To get the pear to lay flat, you can slice a small piece off the back side.
3. Place the agave syrup, currants, walnuts, and cloves in a small bowl and mix well. Set this to the side to be used later.
4. Put the pears on a cookie sheet that has parchment paper on it. Make sure the cored sides are facing up. Sprinkle each pear half with about .5 tablespoon of the chopped walnut mixture.
5. Place into the oven and cook for 25 to 30 minutes. Pears should be tender.

Nutrition : Calories: 103.9; Fiber: 3.1 g; Carbohydrates: 22 g

Butternut Squash Pie

Preparation Time : 25 minutes

Cooking Time : 35 minutes

Servings : 4

Ingredients :

- For the Crust
- Cold water
- Agave, splash
- Sea salt, pinch
- Grapeseed oil, .5 c
- Coconut flour, .5 c
- Spelt Flour, 1 c
- For the Filling
- Butternut squash, peeled, chopped
- Water
- Allspice, to taste
- Agave syrup, to taste
- Hemp milk, 1 c
- Sea moss, 4 tbsp.

Directions :

1. You will need to warm your oven to 350.
2. For the Crust
3. Place the grapeseed oil and water into the refrigerator to get it cold. This will take about one hour.

4. Place all Ingredients into a large bowl. Now you need to add in the cold water a little bit in small amounts until a dough form. Place this onto a surface that has been sprinkled with some coconut flour. Knead for a few minutes and roll the dough as thin as you can get it. Carefully, pick it up and place it inside a pie plate.

5. Place the butternut squash into a Dutch oven and pour in enough water to cover. Bring this to a full rolling boil. Let this cook until the squash has become soft.

6. Completely drain and place into bowl. Using a potato masher, mash the squash. Add in some allspice and agave to taste. Add in the sea moss and hemp milk. Using a hand mixer, blend well. Pour into the pie crust.

7. Place into an oven and bake for about one hour.

Nutrition : Calories: 245; Carbohydrates: 50 g; Fat: 10 g

Coconut Chia Cream Pot

Preparation Time : 5 minutes

Cooking Time : 5 minutes

Servings : 4

Ingredients :

- Date, one (1)
- Coconut milk (organic), one (1) cup
- Coconut yogurt, one (1) cup
- Vanilla extract, ½ teaspoon
- Chia seeds, ¼ cup
- Sesame seeds, one (1) teaspoon
- Flaxseed (ground), one (1) tablespoon or flax meal, one (1) tablespoon
- Toppings:
- Fig, one (1)
- Blueberries, one (1) handful
- Mixed nuts (brazil nuts, almonds, pistachios, macadamia, etc.)
- Cinnamon (ground), one teaspoon

Directions :

1. First, blend the date with coconut milk (the idea is to sweeten the coconut milk).

2. Get a mixing bowl and add the coconut milk with the vanilla, sesame seeds, chia seeds, and flax meal.

3. Refrigerate for between twenty to thirty minutes or wait till the chia expands.

4. To serve, pour a layer of coconut yogurt in a small glass, then add the chia mix, followed by pouring another layer of the coconut yogurt.

5. It's alkaline, creamy and delicious.

Nutrition : Calories: 310; Carbohydrates: 39 g; Protein: 4 g; Fiber: 8.1 g

Chocolate Avocado Mousse

Preparation Time : 10 minutes

Cooking Time : 5 minutes

Servings : 4

Ingredients :

- Coconut water, 2/3 cup
- Avocado, ½ hass
- Raw cacao, 2 teaspoons
- Vanilla, 1 teaspoon
- Dates, three (3)
- Sea salt, one (1) teaspoon
- Dark chocolate shavings

Directions :

1. Blend all Ingredients.
2. Blast until it becomes thick and smooth, as you wish.
3. Put in a fridge and allow it to get firm.

Nutrition : Calories: 181.8; Fat: 151. G; Protein: 12 g

Chia Vanilla Coconut Pudding

Preparation Time : 5 minutes

Cooking Time : 5 minutes

Servings : 2

Ingredients :

- Coconut oil, 2 tablespoons
- Raw cashew, ½ cup
- Coconut water, ½ cup
- Cinnamon, 1 teaspoon
- Dates (pitted), 3
- Vanilla, 2 teaspoons
- Coconut flakes (unsweetened), 1 teaspoon
- Salt (Himalayan or Celtic Grey)
- Chia seeds, 6 tablespoons
- Cinnamon or pomegranate seeds for garnish (optional)

Directions :

1. Get a blender, add all the Ingredients (minus the pomegranate and chia seeds), and blend for about forty to sixty seconds.

2. Reduce the blender speed to the lowest and add the chia seeds.

3. Pour the content into an airtight container and put in a refrigerator for five to six hours.

4. To serve, you can garnish with the cinnamon powder of pomegranate seeds.

Nutrition : Calories: 201; Fat: 10 g; Sodium: 32.8 mg

Sweet Tahini Dip with Ginger Cinnamon Fruit

Preparation Time : 10 minutes

Cooking Time : 5 minutes

Servings : 2

Ingredients :

- Cinnamon, one (1) teaspoon
- Green apple, one (1)
- Pear, one (1)
- Fresh ginger, two (2) – three (3)
- Celtic sea salt, one (1) teaspoon
- Ingredient for sweet Tahini
- Almond butter (raw), three (3) teaspoons
- Tahini (one big scoop), three (3) teaspoons
- Coconut oil, two (2) teaspoons
- Cayenne (optional), ¼ teaspoons
- Wheat-free tamari, two (2) teaspoons
- Liquid coconut nectar, one (1) teaspoon

Directions :

1. Get a clean mixing bowl.
2. Grate the ginger, add cinnamon, sea salt and mix together in the bowl.
3. Dice apple and pear into little cubes, turn into the bowl and mix.
4. Get a mixing bowl and mix all the Ingredients.

5. Then add the Sprinkle the Sweet Tahini Dip all over the Ginger Cinnamon Fruit.

6. Serve.

Nutrition : Calories: 109; Fat: 10.8 g; Sodium: 258 mg

Coconut Butter and Chopped Berries with Mint

Preparation Time : 5 minutes

Cooking Time : 5 minutes

Servings : 4

Ingredients :

- Chopped mint, one (1) tablespoon

- Coconut butter (melted), two (2) tablespoons

- Mixed berries (strawberries, blueberries, and raspberries)

Directions :

1. Get a small bowl and add the berries.

2. Drizzle the melted coconut butter and sprinkle the mint.

3. Serve.

Nutrition : Calories: 159; Fat: 12 g; Carbohydrates: 18 g

Alkaline Raw Pumpkin Pie

Preparation Time : 5 minutes

Cooking Time : 5 minutes

Servings : 4

Ingredients :

Ingredients for Pie Crust

- Cinnamon, one (1) teaspoon
- Dates/Turkish apricots, one (1) cup
- Raw almonds, one (1) cup
- Coconut flakes (unsweetened), one (1) cup

Ingredients for Pie Filling

- Dates, six (6)
- Cinnamon, ½ teaspoon
- Nutmeg, ½ teaspoon
- Pecans (soaked overnight), one (1) cup
- Organic pumpkin Blends (12 oz.), 1 ¼ cup
- Nutmeg, ½ teaspoon
- Sea salt (Himalayan or Celtic Sea Salt), ¼ teaspoon
- Vanilla, 1 teaspoon
- Gluten-free tamari

Directions :

Directions for pie crust

1. Get a food processor and blend all the pie crust Ingredients at the same time.

2. Make sure the mixture turns oily and sticky before you stop mixing.

3. Put the mixture in a pie pan and mold against the sides and floor, to make it stick properly.

Directions for the pie filling

1. Mix Ingredients together in a blender.

2. Add the mixture to fill in the pie crust.

3. Pour some cinnamon on top.

4. Then refrigerate till it's cold.

5. Then mold.

Nutrition : Calories 135; Calories from Fat 41.4; Total Fat 4.6 g; Cholesterol 11.3 mg

Strawberry Sorbet

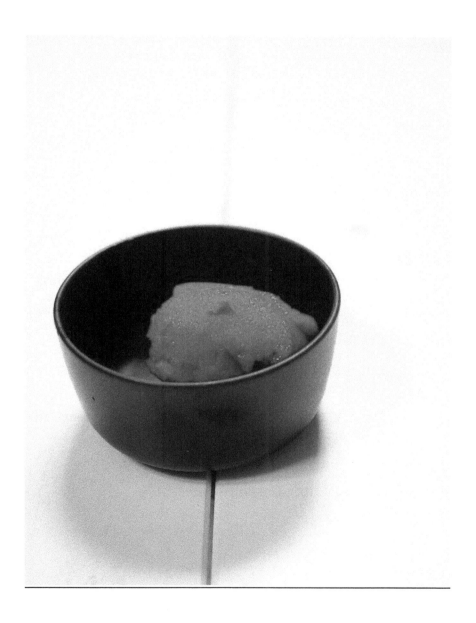

Preparation Time : 5 minutes

Cooking Time : 4 Hours

Servings : 4

Ingredients :

- 2 cups of Strawberries*
- 1 1/2 teaspoons of Spelt Flour
- 1/2 cup of Date Sugar
- 2 cups of Spring Water

Directions :

- Add Date Sugar, Spring Water, and Spelt Flour to a medium pot and boil on low heat for about ten minutes. Mixture should thicken, like syrup.
- Remove the pot from the heat and allow it to cool.
- After cooling, add Blend Strawberry and mix gently.
- Put mixture in a container and freeze.
- Cut it into pieces, put the sorbet into a processor and blend until smooth.
- Put everything back in the container and leave in the refrigerator for at least four hours.
- Serve and enjoy your Strawberry Sorbet!

Nutrition : Calories: 198; Carbohydrates: 28 g

Blueberry Muffins

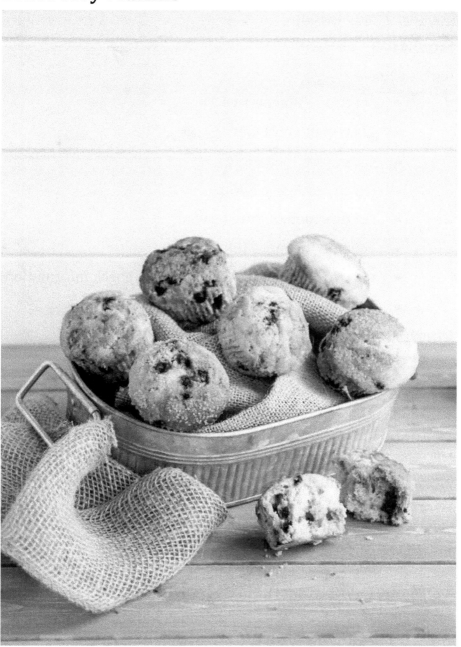

Preparation Time : 5 minutes

Cooking Time : 1 Hour

Servings : 3

Ingredients :

- 1/2 cup of Blueberries
- 3/4 cup of Teff Flour
- 3/4 cup of Spelt Flour
- 1/3 cup of Agave Syrup
- 1/2 teaspoon of Pure Sea Salt
- 1 cup of Coconut Milk
- 1/4 cup of Sea Moss Gel (optional, check information)
- Grape Seed Oil

Directions :

1. Preheat your oven to 365 degrees Fahrenheit.
2. Grease or line 6 standard muffin cups.
3. Add Teff, Spelt flour, Pure Sea Salt, Coconut Milk, Sea Moss Gel, and Agave Syrup to a large bowl. Mix them together.
4. Add Blueberries to the mixture and mix well.
5. Divide muffin batter among the 6 muffin cups.
6. Bake for 30 minutes until golden brown.
7. Serve and enjoy your Blueberry Muffins!

Nutrition : Calories: 65; Fat: 0.7 g; Carbohydrates: 12 g; Protein: 1.4 g; Fiber: 5 g

Banana Strawberry Ice Cream

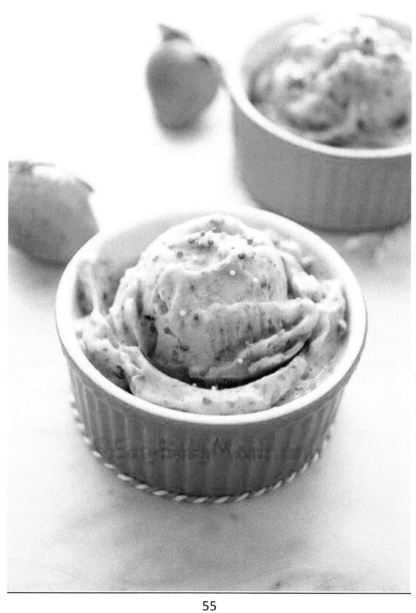

Preparation Time : 5 minutes

Cooking Time : 4 Hours

Servings : 5

Ingredients :

- 1 cup of Strawberry*
- 5 quartered Baby Bananas*
- 1/2 Avocado, chopped
- 1 tablespoon of Agave Syrup
- 1/4 cup of Homemade Walnut Milk

Directions :

1. Mix Ingredients into the blender and blend them well.
2. Taste. If it is too thick, add extra Milk or Agave Syrup if you want it sweeter.
3. Put in a container with a lid and allow to freeze for at least 5 to 6 hours.
4. Serve it and enjoy your Banana Strawberry Ice Cream!

Nutrition : Calories: 200; Fat: 0.5 g; Carbohydrates: 44 g

Homemade Whipped Cream

Preparation Time : 5 minutes

Cooking Time : 10 Minutes

Servings : 1 Cup

Ingredients :

- 1 cup of Aquafaba
- 1/4 cup of Agave Syrup

Directions :

1. Add Agave Syrup and Aquafaba into a bowl.
2. Mix at high speed around 5 minutes with a stand mixer or 10 to 15 minutes with a hand mixer.
3. Serve and enjoy your Homemade Whipped Cream!

Nutrition : Calories: 21; Fat: 0g; Sodium: 0.3g; Carbohydrates: 5.3g; Fiber: 0g; Sugars: 4.7g; Protein: 0g

Chocolate Crunch Bars

Preparation Time : 5 minutes

Cooking Time : 5 minutes

Servings : 4

Ingredients :

- 1 1/2 cups sugar-free chocolate chips
- 1 cup almond butter
- Stevia to taste
- 1/4 cup coconut oil
- 3 cups pecans, chopped

Directions :

1. Layer an 8-inch baking pan with parchment paper.
2. Mix chocolate chips with butter, coconut oil, and sweetener in a bowl.
3. Melt it by heating in a microwave for 2 to 3 minutes until well mixed.
4. Stir in nuts and seeds. Mix gently.
5. Pour this batter carefully into the baking pan and spread evenly.
6. Refrigerate for 2 to 3 hours.
7. Slice and serve.

Nutrition : Calories 316; Total Fat 30.9 g; Saturated Fat 8.1 g; Cholesterol 0 mg; Total Carbs 8.3 g; Sugar 1.8 g; Fiber 3.8 g; Sodium 8 mg; Protein 6.4 g

Homemade Protein Bar

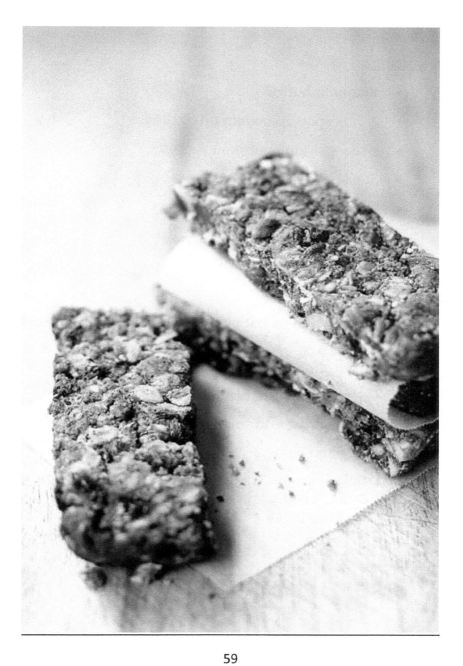

Preparation Time : 5 minutes

Cooking Time : 10 minutes

Servings : 4

Ingredients :

- 1 cup nut butter
- 4 tablespoons coconut oil
- 2 scoops vanilla protein
- Stevia, to taste
- ½ teaspoon sea salt
- Optional Ingredients
- 1 teaspoon cinnamon

Directions:

1. Mix coconut oil with butter, protein, stevia, and salt in a dish.
2. Stir in cinnamon and chocolate chip.
3. Press the mixture firmly and freeze until firm.
4. Cut the crust into small bars.
5. Serve and enjoy.

Nutrition : Calories 179; Total Fat 15.7 g; Saturated Fat 8 g; Cholesterol 0 mg; Total Carbs 4.8 g; Sugar 3.6 g; Fiber 0.8 g; Sodium 43 mg; Protein 5.6 g

Shortbread Cookies

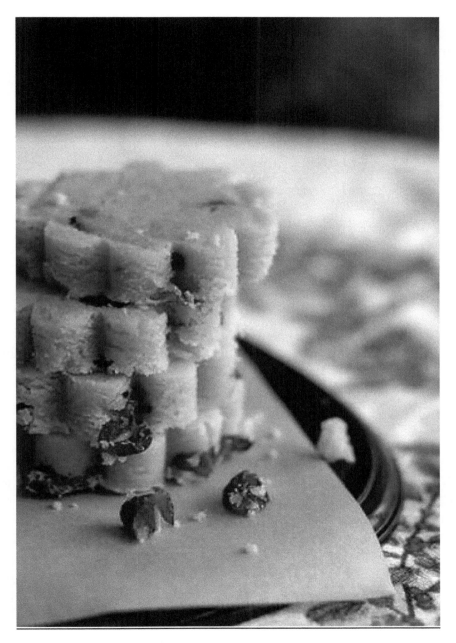

Preparation Time : 10 minutes

Cooking Time : 70 minutes

Servings : 6

Ingredients :

- 2 1/2 cups almond flour
- 6 tablespoons nut butter
- 1/2 cup erythritol
- 1 teaspoon vanilla essence

Directions :

1. Preheat your oven to 350 degrees F.
2. Layer a cookie sheet with parchment paper.
3. Beat butter with erythritol until fluffy.
4. Stir in vanilla essence and almond flour. Mix well until becomes crumbly.
5. Spoon out a tablespoon of cookie dough onto the cookie sheet.
6. Add more dough to make as many cookies.
7. Bake for 15 minutes until brown.
8. Serve.

Nutrition : Calories 288; Total Fat 25.3 g; Saturated Fat 6.7 g; Cholesterol 23 mg; Total Carbs 9.6 g; Sugar 0.1 g; Fiber 3.8 g; Sodium 74 mg; Potassium 3 mg; Protein 7.6 g

Coconut Chip Cookies

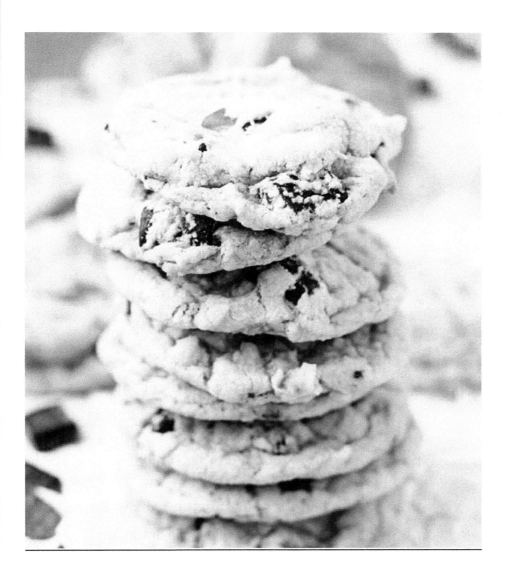

Preparation Time : 10 minutes

Cooking Time : 15 minutes

Servings : 4

Ingredients :

- 1 cup almond flour
- ½ cup cacao nibs
- ½ cup coconut flakes, unsweetened
- 1/3 cup erythritol
- ½ cup almond butter
- ¼ cup nut butter, melted
- ¼ cup almond milk
- Stevia, to taste
- ¼ teaspoon sea salt

Directions :

1. Preheat your oven to 350 degrees F.
2. Layer a cookie sheet with parchment paper.
3. Add and then combine all the dry Ingredients in a glass bowl.
4. Whisk in butter, almond milk, vanilla essence, stevia, and almond butter.
5. Beat well then stir in dry mixture. Mix well.
6. Spoon out a tablespoon of cookie dough on the cookie sheet.
7. Add more dough to make as many as 16 cookies.
8. Flatten each cookie using your fingers.

9. Bake for 25 minutes until golden brown.

10. Let them sit for 15 minutes.

11. Serve.

Nutrition : Calories 192; Total Fat 17.44 g; Saturated Fat 11.5 g; Cholesterol 125 mg; Total Carbs 2.2 g; Sugar 1.4 g; Fiber 2.1 g; Sodium 135 mg; Protein 4.7 g

Peanut Butter Cups

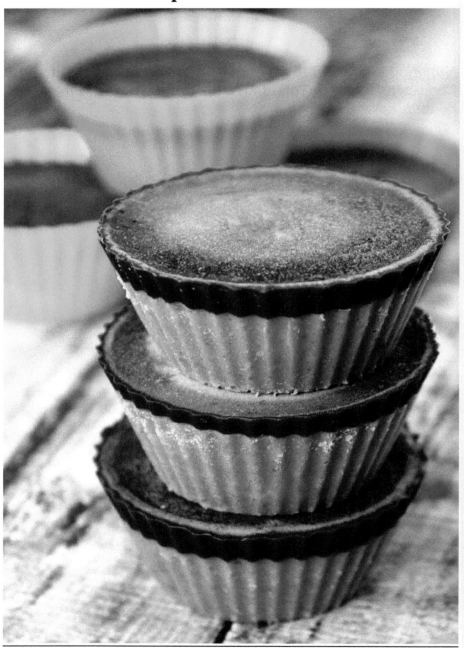

Preparation Time : 5 minutes

Cooking Time : 10 minutes

Servings : 4

Ingredients :

- 1 packet plain gelatin
- ¼ cup sugar substitute
- 2 cups nonfat cream
- ½ teaspoon vanilla
- ¼ cup low-fat peanut butter
- 2 tablespoons unsalted peanuts, chopped

Directions :

1. Mix gelatin, sugar substitute and cream in a pan.
2. Let sit for 5 minutes.
3. Place over medium heat and cook until gelatin has been dissolved.
4. Stir in vanilla and peanut butter.
5. Pour into custard cups. Chill for 3 hours.
6. Top with the peanuts and serve.

Nutrition : 171 Calories; 21g Carbohydrate; 6.8g Protein

Fruit Pizza

Preparation Time : 5 minutes

Cooking Time : 10 minutes

Servings : 4

Ingredients :

- 1 teaspoon maple syrup
- ¼ teaspoon vanilla extract
- ½ cup coconut milk yogurt
- 2 round slices watermelon
- ½ cup blackberries, sliced
- ½ cup strawberries, sliced
- 2 tablespoons coconut flakes (unsweetened)

Directions :

1. Mix maple syrup, vanilla and yogurt in a bowl.
2. Spread the mixture on top of the watermelon slice.
3. Top with the berries and coconut flakes.

Nutrition : 70 Calories; 14.6g Carbohydrate; 1.2g Protein

Choco Peppermint Cake

Preparation Time : 5 minutes

Cooking Time : 10 minutes

Servings : 4

Ingredients :

- Cooking spray
- 1/3 cup oil
- 15 oz. package chocolate cake mix
- 3 eggs, beaten
- 1 cup water
- ¼ teaspoon peppermint extract

Directions :

1. Spray slow cooker with oil.
2. Mix all the ingredients in a bowl.
3. Use an electric mixer on medium speed setting to mix ingredients for 2 minutes.
4. Pour mixture into the slow cooker.
5. Cover the pot and cook on low for 3 hours.
6. Let cool before slicing and serving.

Nutrition : 185 Calories; 27g Carbohydrate; 3.8g Protein

Roasted Mango

Preparation Time : 5 minutes

Cooking Time : 10 minutes

Servings : 4

Ingredients :

- 2 mangoes, sliced
- 2 teaspoons crystallized ginger, chopped
- 2 teaspoons orange zest
- 2 tablespoons coconut flakes (unsweetened)

Directions :

1. Preheat your oven to 350 degrees F.
2. Add mango slices in custard cups.
3. Top with the ginger, orange zest and coconut flakes.
4. Bake in the oven for 10 minutes.

Nutrition : 89 Calories; 20g Carbohydrate; 0.8g Protein

Roasted Plums

Preparation Time : 5 minutes

Cooking Time : 10 minutes

Servings : 4

Ingredients :

- Cooking spray
- 6 plums, sliced
- ½ cup pineapple juice (unsweetened)
- 1 tablespoon brown sugar
- 2 tablespoons brown sugar
- ¼ teaspoon ground cardamom
- ½ teaspoon ground cinnamon
- 1/8 teaspoon ground cumin

Directions :

1. Combine all the ingredients in a baking pan.
2. Roast in the oven at 450 degrees F for 20 minutes.

Nutrition : 102 Calories; 18.7g Carbohydrate; 2g Protein

Figs with Honey & Yogurt

Preparation Time : 5 minutes

Cooking Time : 10 minutes

Servings : 4

Ingredients :

- ½ teaspoon vanilla
- 8 oz. nonfat yogurt
- 2 figs, sliced
- 1 tablespoon walnuts, chopped and toasted
- 2 teaspoons honey

Directions :

1. Stir vanilla into yogurt.
2. Mix well.
3. Top with the figs and sprinkle with walnuts.
4. Drizzle with honey and serve.

Nutrition : 157 Calories; 24g Carbohydrate; 7g Protein

Flourless Chocolate Cake

Preparation Time : 10 minutes

Cooking Time : 45 minutes

Servings : 6

Ingredients :

- ½ Cup of stevia
- 12 Ounces of unsweetened baking chocolate
- 2/3 Cup of ghee
- 1/3 Cup of warm water
- ¼ Teaspoon of salt
- 4 Large pastured eggs
- 2 Cups of boiling water

Directions :

1. Line the bottom of a 9-inch pan of a spring form with a parchment paper.

2. Heat the water in a small pot; then add the salt and the stevia over the water until wait until the mixture becomes completely dissolved.

3. Melt the baking chocolate into a double boiler or simply microwave it for about 30 seconds.

4. Mix the melted chocolate and the butter in a large bowl with an electric mixer.

5. Beat in your hot mixture; then crack in the egg and whisk after adding each of the eggs.

6. Pour the obtained mixture into your prepared spring form tray.

7. Wrap the spring form tray with a foil paper.

8. Place the spring form tray in a large cake tray and add boiling water right to the outside; make sure the depth doesn't exceed 1 inch.

9. Bake the cake into the water bath for about 45 minutes at a temperature of about 350 F.

10. Remove the tray from the boiling water and transfer to a wire to cool.

11. Let the cake chill for an overnight in the refrigerator.

Nutrition: 295 Calories; 6g Carbohydrates; 4g Fiber

Lava Cake

Preparation Time : 10 minutes

Cooking Time : 10 minutes

Servings : 2

Ingredients :

- 2 Oz of dark chocolate; you should at least use chocolate of 85% cocoa solids
- 1 Tablespoon of super-fine almond flour
- 2 Oz of unsalted almond butter
- 2 Large eggs

Directions :

1. Heat your oven to a temperature of about 350 Fahrenheit.
2. Grease 2 heat proof ramekins with almond butter.
3. Now, melt the chocolate and the almond butter and stir very well.
4. Beat the eggs very well with a mixer.
5. Add the eggs to the chocolate and the butter mixture and mix very well with almond flour and the swerve; then stir.
6. Pour the dough into 2 ramekins.
7. Bake for about 9 to 10 minutes.
8. Turn the cakes over plates and serve with pomegranate seeds!

Nutrition: 459 Calories; 3.5g Carbohydrates; 0.8g Fiber

Cheese Cake

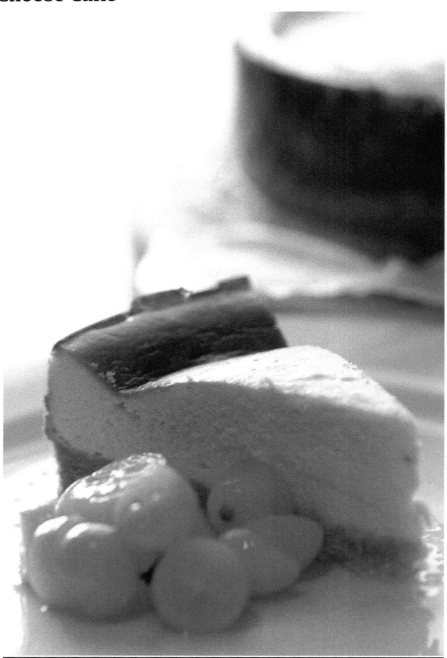

Preparation Time : 15 minutes

Cooking Time : 50 minutes

Servings : 6

Ingredients :

For Almond Flour Cheesecake Crust:

- 2 Cups of Blanched almond flour
- 1/3 Cup of almond Butter
- 3 Tablespoons of Erythritol (powdered or granular)
- 1 Teaspoon of Vanilla extract

For Keto Cheesecake Filling:

- 32 Oz of softened Cream cheese
- 1 and ¼ cups of powdered erythritol
- 3 Large Eggs
- 1 Tablespoon of Lemon juice
- 1 Teaspoon of Vanilla extract

Directions :

1. Preheat your oven to a temperature of about 350 degrees F.
2. Grease a spring form pan of 9¨ with cooking spray or just line its bottom with a parchment paper.
3. In order to make the cheesecake rust, stir in the melted butter, the almond flour, the vanilla extract and the erythritol in a large bowl.
4. The dough will get will be a bit crumbly; so, press it into the bottom of your prepared tray.

5. Bake for about 12 minutes; then let cool for about 10 minutes.

6. In the meantime, beat the softened cream cheese and the powdered sweetener at a low speed until it becomes smooth.

7. Crack in the eggs and beat them in at a low to medium speed until it becomes fluffy. Make sure to add one a time.

8. Add in the lemon juice and the vanilla extract and mix at a low to medium speed with a mixer.

9. Pour your filling into your pan right on top of the crust. You can use a spatula to smooth the top of the cake.

10. Bake for about 45 to 50 minutes.

11. Remove the baked cheesecake from your oven and run a knife around its edge.

12. Let the cake cool for about 4 hours in the refrigerator.

13. Serve and enjoy your delicious cheese cake!

Nutrition: 325 Calories; 6g Carbohydrates; 1g Fiber

Orange Cake

Preparation Time : 10 minutes

Cooking Time : 50minutes

Servings : 8

Ingredients :

- 2 and ½ cups of almond flour
- 2 Unwaxed washed oranges
- 5 Large separated eggs
- 1 Teaspoon of baking powder
- 2 Teaspoons of orange extract
- 1 Teaspoon of vanilla bean powder
- 6 Seeds of cardamom pods crushed
- 16 drops of liquid stevia; about 3 teaspoons
- 1 Handful of flaked almonds to decorate

Directions :

1. Preheat your oven to a temperature of about 350 Fahrenheit.
2. Line a rectangular bread baking tray with a parchment paper.
3. Place the oranges into a pan filled with cold water and cover it with a lid.
4. Bring the saucepan to a boil, then let simmer for about 1 hour and make sure the oranges are totally submerged.
5. Make sure the oranges are always submerged to remove any taste of bitterness.

6. Cut the oranges into halves; then remove any seeds; and drain the water and set the oranges aside to cool down.

7. Cut the oranges in half and remove any seeds, then puree it with a blender or a food processor.

8. Separate the eggs; then whisk the egg whites until you see stiff peaks forming.

9. Add all your ingredients except for the egg whites to the orange mixture and add in the egg whites; then mix.

10. Pour the batter into the cake tin and sprinkle with the flaked almonds right on top.

11. Bake your cake for about 50 minutes.

12. Remove the cake from the oven and set aside to cool for 5 minutes.

Nutrition: 164 Calories; 7.1g Carbohydrates; 2.7g Fiber

Madeleine

Preparation Time : 10 minutes

Cooking Time : 15 minutes

Servings : 12

Ingredients :

- 2 Large pastured eggs
- ¾ Cup of almond flour
- 1 and ½ Tablespoons of Swerve
- ¼ Cup of cooled, melted coconut oil
- 1 Teaspoon of vanilla extract
- 1 Teaspoon of almond extract
- 1 Teaspoon of lemon zest
- ¼ Teaspoon of salt

Directions:

1. Preheat your oven to a temperature of about 350 F.
2. Combine the eggs with the salt and whisk on a high speed for about 5 minutes.
3. Slowly add in the Swerve and keep mixing on high for 2 additional minutes.
4. Stir in the almond flour until it is very well-incorporated; then add in the vanilla and the almond extracts.
5. Add in the melted coconut oil and stir all your ingredients together.
6. Pour the obtained batter into equal parts in a greased Madeleine tray.

7. Bake your Ketogenic Madeleine for about 13 minutes or until the edges start to have a brown color.

8. Flip the Madeleines out of the baking tray.

Nutrition: 87 Calories; 3g Carbohydrates; 3g Fiber

Waffles

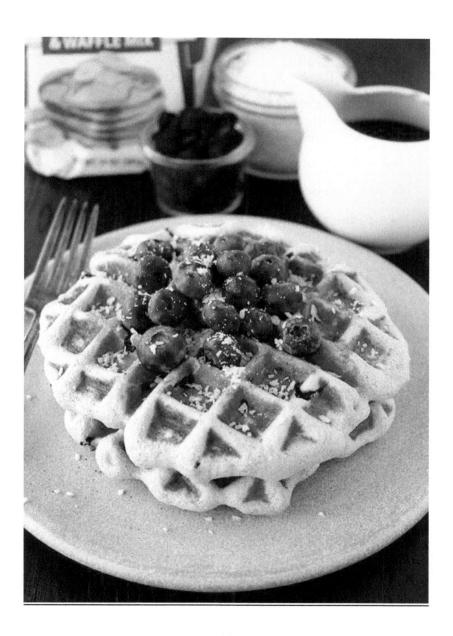

Preparation Time : 20 minutes

Cooking Time : 30 minutes

Servings : 3

Ingredients :

For Ketogenic waffles:

- 8 Oz of cream cheese
- 5 Large pastured eggs
- 1/3 Cup of coconut flour
- ½ Teaspoon of Xanthan gum
- 1 Pinch of salt
- ½ Teaspoon of vanilla extract
- 2 Tablespoons of Swerve
- ¼ Teaspoon of baking soda
- 1/3 Cup of almond milk

Optional ingredients:

- ½ Teaspoon of cinnamon pie spice
- ¼ Teaspoon of almond extract

For low-carb Maple Syrup:

- 1 Cup of water
- 1 Tablespoon of Maple flavor
- ¾ Cup of powdered Swerve
- 1 Tablespoon of almond butter
- ½ Teaspoon of Xanthan gum

Directions:

For the waffles:

1. Make sure all your ingredients are exactly at room temperature.

2. Place all your ingredients for the waffles from cream cheese to pastured eggs, coconut flour, Xanthan gum, salt, vanilla extract, the Swerve, the baking soda and the almond milk except for the almond milk with the help of a processor.

3. Blend your ingredients until it becomes smooth and creamy; then transfer the batter to a bowl.

4. Add the almond milk and mix your ingredients with a spatula.

5. Heat a waffle maker to a temperature of high.

6. Spray your waffle maker with coconut oil and add about ¼ of the batter in it evenly with a spatula into your waffle iron.

7. Close your waffle and cook until you get the color you want.

8. Carefully remove the waffles to a platter.

For the Ketogenic Maple Syrup:

9. Place 1 and ¼ cups of water, the swerve and the maple in a small pan and bring to a boil over a low heat; then let simmer for about 10 minutes.

10. Add the coconut oil.

11. Sprinkle the Xanthan gum over the top of the waffle and use an immersion blender to blend smoothly.

12. Serve and enjoy your delicious waffles!

Nutrition: 316 Calories; 7g Carbohydrates; 3g Fiber

Pretzels

Preparation Time : 10 minutes

Cooking Time : 20 minutes

Servings : 8

Ingredients :

- 1 and ½ cups of pre-shredded mozzarella
- 2 Tablespoons of full fat cream cheese
- 1 Large egg
- ¾ Cup of almond flour+ 2 tablespoons of ground almonds or almond meal
- ½ Teaspoon of baking powder
- 1 Pinch of coarse sea salt

Directions :

1. Heat your oven to a temperature of about 180 C/356 F.

2. Melt the cream cheese and the mozzarella cheese and stir over a low heat until the cheeses are perfectly melted.

3. If you choose to microwave the cheese, just do that for about 1 minute no more and if you want to do it on the stove, turn off the heat as soon as the cheese is completely melted.

4. Add the large egg to the prepared warm dough; then stir until your ingredients are very well combined. If the egg is cold; you will need to heat it gently.

5. Add in the ground almonds or the almond flour and the baking powder and stir until your ingredients are very well combined.

6. Take one pinch of the dough of cheese and toll it or stretch it in your hands until it is about 18 to 20 cm of length; if your dough is sticky, you can oil your hands to avoid that.

7. Now, form pretzels from the cheese dough and nicely shape it; then place it over a baking sheet.

8. Sprinkle with a little bit of salt and bake for about 17 minutes.

Nutrition: 113 Calories; 2.5g Carbohydrates; 0.8g Fiber

Cheesy Taco Bites

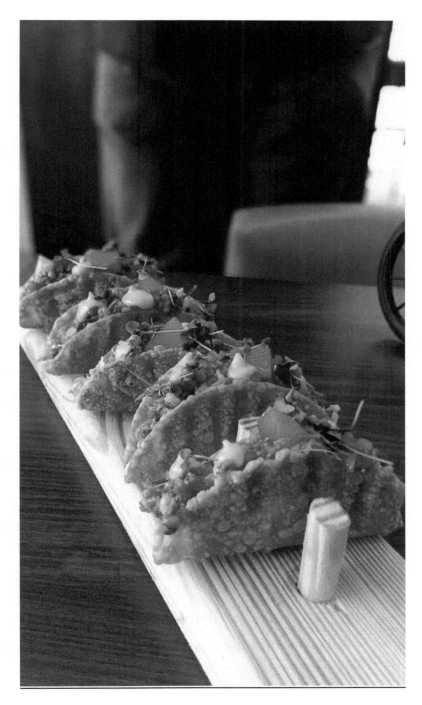

Preparation Time : 5 minutes

Cooking Time : 10minutes

Serving : 12

Ingredients:

- 2 Cups of Packaged Shredded Cheddar Cheese
- 2 Tablespoon of Chili Powder
- 2 Tablespoons of Cumin
- 1 Teaspoon of Salt
- 8 Teaspoons of coconut cream for garnishing
- Use Pico de Gallo for garnishing as well

Directions :

1. Preheat your oven to a temperature of about 350 F.

2. Over a baking sheet lined with a parchment paper, place 1 tablespoon piles of cheese and make sure to a space of 2 inches between each.

3. Place the baking sheet in your oven and bake for about 5 minutes.

4. Remove from the oven and let the cheese cool down for about 1 minute; then carefully lift up and press each into the cups of a mini muffin tin.

5. Make sure to press the edges of the cheese to form the shape of muffins mini.

6. Let the cheese cool completely; then remove it.

7. While you continue to bake the cheese and create your cups.

8. Fill the cheese cups with the coconut cream, then top with the Pico de Gallo.

Nutrition: 73 Calories; 3g Carbohydrates; 4g Protein

Nut Squares

Preparation Time : 30 minutes

Cooking Time : 10 minutes

Serving : 10

Ingredients :

- 2 Cups of almonds, pumpkin seeds, sunflower seeds and walnuts
- ½ Cup of desiccated coconut
- 1 Tablespoon of chia seeds
- ¼ Teaspoon of salt
- 2 Tablespoons of coconut oil
- 1 Teaspoon of vanilla extract
- 3 Tablespoons of almond or peanut butter
- 1/3 Cup of Sukrin Gold Fiber Syrup

Directions :

1. Line a square baking tin with a baking paper; then lightly grease it with cooking spray
2. Chop all the nuts roughly; then slightly grease it too, you can also leave them as whole
3. Mix the nuts in a large bowl; then combine them in a large bowl with the coconut, the chia seeds and the salt
4. In a microwave-proof bowl; add the coconut oil; then add the vanilla, the coconut butter or oil, the almond butter and the fiber syrup and microwave the mixture for about 30 seconds
5. Stir your ingredients together very well; then pour the melted mixture right on top of the nuts

6. Press the mixture into your prepared baking tin with the help of the back of a measuring cup and push very well

7. Freeze your treat for about 1 hour before cutting it

8. Cut your frozen nut batter into small cubes or squares of the same size

Nutrition: 268 Calories; 14g Carbohydrates; 1g Fiber

Pumpkin & Banana Ice Cream

Preparation Time : 5 minutes

Cooking Time : 10 minutes

Servings : 4

Ingredients :

- 15 oz. pumpkin puree
- 4 bananas, sliced and frozen
- 1 teaspoon pumpkin pie spice
- Chopped pecans

Directions :

1. Add pumpkin puree, bananas and pumpkin pie spice in a food processor.
2. Pulse until smooth.
3. Chill in the refrigerator.
4. Garnish with pecans.

Nutrition : 71 Calories 18g; Carbohydrate; 1.2g Protein

Brulee Oranges

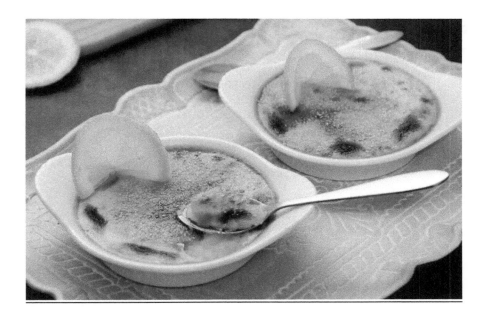

Preparation Time : 5 minutes

Cooking Time : 10 minutes

Servings : 4

Ingredients :

- 4 oranges, sliced into segments
- 1 teaspoon ground cardamom
- 6 teaspoons brown sugar
- 1 cup nonfat Greek yogurt

Directions :

1. Preheat your broiler.
2. Arrange orange slices in a baking pan.
3. In a bowl, mix the cardamom and sugar.
4. Sprinkle mixture on top of the oranges. Broil for 5 minutes.
5. Serve oranges with yogurt.

Nutrition : 168 Calories; 26.9g Carbohydrate; 6.8g Protein

Frozen Lemon & Blueberry

Preparation Time : 5 minutes

Cooking Time : 10 minutes

Servings : 4

Ingredients :

- 6 cup fresh blueberries
- 8 sprigs fresh thyme
- ¾ cup light brown sugar
- 1 teaspoon lemon zest
- ¼ cup lemon juice
- 2 cups water

Directions :

1. Add blueberries, thyme and sugar in a pan over medium heat.
2. Cook for 6 to 8 minutes.
3. Transfer mixture to a blender.
4. Remove thyme sprigs.
5. Stir in the remaining ingredients.
6. Pulse until smooth.
7. Strain mixture and freeze for 1 hour.

Nutrition : 78 Calories; 20g Carbohydrate; 3g Protein

Peanut Butter Choco Chip Cookies

Preparation Time : 5 minutes

Cooking Time : 10 minutes

Servings : 4

Ingredients :

- 1 egg
- ½ cup light brown sugar
- 1 cup natural unsweetened peanut butter
- Pinch salt
- ¼ cup dark chocolate chips

Directions :

1. Preheat your oven to 375 degrees F.
2. Mix egg, sugar, peanut butter, salt and chocolate chips in a bowl.
3. Form into cookies and place in a baking pan.
4. Bake the cookie for 10 minutes.
5. Let cool before serving.

Nutrition : 159 Calories; 12g Carbohydrate; 4.3g Protein

Watermelon Sherbet

Preparation Time : 5 minutes

Cooking Time : 3 minutes

Servings : 4

Ingredients :

- 6 cups watermelon, sliced into cubes
- 14 oz. almond milk
- 1 tablespoon honey
- ¼ cup lime juice
- Salt to taste

Directions :

1. Freeze watermelon for 4 hours.
2. Add frozen watermelon and other ingredients in a blender.
3. Blend until smooth.
4. Transfer to a container with seal.
5. Seal and freeze for 4 hours.

Nutrition : 132 Calories; 24.5g Carbohydrate; 3.1g Protein

Strawberry & Mango Ice Cream

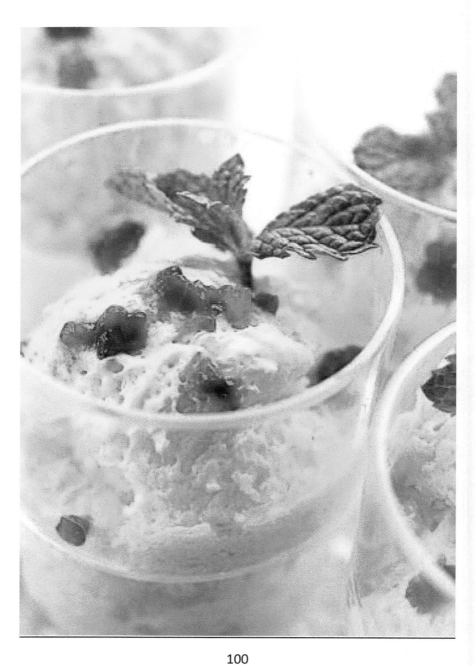

Preparation Time : 5 minutes

Cooking Time : 10 minutes

Servings : 4

Ingredients :

- 8 oz. strawberries, sliced
- 12 oz. mango, sliced into cubes
- 1 tablespoon lime juice

Directions :

1. Add all ingredients in a food processor.
2. Pulse for 2 minutes.
3. Chill before serving.

Nutrition : 70 Calories; 17.4g Carbohydrate; 1.1g Protein

Sparkling Fruit Drink

Preparation Time : 5 minutes

Cooking Time : 10 minutes

Servings : 4

Ingredients :

- 8 oz. unsweetened grape juice
- 8 oz. unsweetened apple juice
- 8 oz. unsweetened orange juice
- 1 qt. homemade ginger ale
- Ice

Directions :

1. Makes 7 servings. Mix first 4 ingredients together in a pitcher. Stir in ice cubes and 9 ounces of the beverage to each glass. Serve immediately.

Nutrition : 60 Calories; 1.1g Protein

Tiramisu Shots

Preparation Time : 5 minutes

Cooking Time : 10 minutes

Servings : 4

Ingredients :

- 1 pack silken tofu
- 1 oz. dark chocolate, finely chopped
- ¼ cup sugar substitute
- 1 teaspoon lemon juice
- ¼ cup brewed espresso
- Pinch salt
- 24 slices angel food cake
- Cocoa powder (unsweetened)

Directions :

2. Add tofu, chocolate, sugar substitute, lemon juice, espresso and salt in a food processor.
3. Pulse until smooth.
4. Add angel food cake pieces into shot glasses.
5. Drizzle with the cocoa powder.
6. Pour the tofu mixture on top.
7. Top with the remaining angel food cake pieces.
8. Chill for 30 minutes and serve.

Nutrition: 75 Calories; 12g Carbohydrate; 2.9g Protein

Ice Cream Brownie Cake

Preparation Time : 5 minutes

Cooking Time : 10 minutes

Servings : 4

Ingredients :

- Cooking spray
- 12 oz. no-sugar brownie mix
- ¼ cup oil
- 2 egg whites
- 3 tablespoons water
- 2 cups sugar-free ice cream

Directions :

1. Preheat your oven to 325 degrees F.
2. Spray your baking pan with oil.
3. Mix brownie mix, oil, egg whites and water in a bowl.
4. Pour into the baking pan.
5. Bake for 25 minutes.
6. Let cool.
7. Freeze brownie for 2 hours.
8. Spread ice cream over the brownie.
9. Freeze for 8 hours.

Nutrition : 198 Calories; 33g Carbohydrate; 3g Protein

Berry Sorbet

Preparation Time : 10 minutes

Cooking Time : 20 minutes

Servings : 6

Ingredients :

- Water, 2 c
- Blend strawberries, 2 c
- Spelt Flour, 1.5 tsp.
- Date sugar, .5 c

Directions :

1. Add the water into a large pot and let the water begin to warm. Add the flour and date sugar and stir until dissolved. Allow this mixture to start boiling and continue to cook for around ten minutes. It should have started to thicken. Take off the heat and set to the side to cool.

2. Once the syrup has cooled off, add in the strawberries, and stir well to combine.

3. Pour into a container that is freezer safe and put it into the freezer until frozen.

4. Take sorbet out of the freezer, cut into chunks, and put it either into a blender or a food processor. Hit the pulse button until the mixture is creamy.

5. Pour this into the same freezer-safe container and put it back into the freezer for four hours.

Nutrition : Calories: 99; Carbohydrates: 8 g

Quinoa Porridge

Preparation Time : 5 minutes

Cooking Time : 15 minutes

Servings : 4

Ingredients :

- Zest of one lime
- Coconut milk, .5 c
- Cloves, .5 tsp.
- Ground ginger, 1.5 tsp.
- Spring water, 2 c
- Quinoa, 1 c
- Grated apple, 1

Directions :

1. Cook the quinoa. Follow the instructions on the package. When the quinoa has been cooked, drain well. Place it back into the pot and stir in spices.

2. Add coconut milk and stir well to combine.

3. Grate the apple now and stir well.

4. Divide equally into bowls and add the lime zest on top. Sprinkle with nuts and seeds of choice.

Nutrition : Calories: 180; Fat: 3 g; Carbohydrates: 40 g; Protein: 10 g

Apple Quinoa

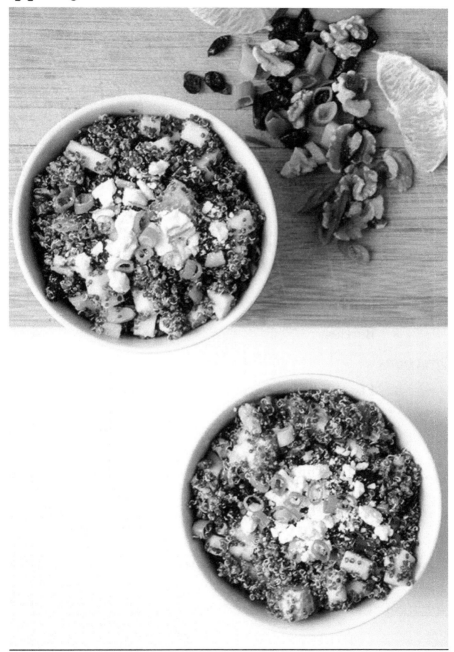

Preparation Time : 15 minutes

Cooking Time : 30 minutes

Servings : 04

Ingredients :

- Coconut oil, 1 tbsp.
- Ginger
- Key lime .5
- Apple, 1
- Quinoa, .5 c
- Optional toppings
- Seeds
- Nuts
- Berries

Directions :

1. Fix the quinoa according to the instructions on the package. When you are getting close to the end of the Cooking time, grate in the apple and cook for 30 seconds.

2. Zest the lime into the quinoa and squeeze the juice in. Stir in the coconut oil.

3. Divide evenly into bowls and sprinkle with some ginger.

4. You can add in some berries, nuts, and seeds right before you eat.

Nutrition : Calories: 146; Fiber: 2.3 g; Fat: 8.3 g

Kamut Porridge

Preparation Time : 10 minutes

Cooking Time : 25 minutes

Servings : 4

Ingredients :

- Agave syrup, 4 tbsp.
- Coconut oil, 1 tbsp.
- Sea salt, .5 tsp.
- Coconut milk, 3.75 c
- Kamut berries, 1 c
- Optional toppings
- Berries
- Coconut chips
- Ground nutmeg
- Ground cloves

Directions :

1. You need to "crack" the Kamut berries. You can try this by placing the berries into a food processor and pulsing until you have 1.25 cups of Kamut.

2. Place the cracked Kamut in a pot with salt and coconut milk. Give it a good stir in order to combine everything. Allow this mixture to come to a full rolling boil and then turn the heat down until the mixture is simmering. Stir every now and then until the Kamut has thickened to your likeness. This normally takes about ten minutes.

3. Take off heat, stir in agave syrup and coconut oil.

4. Garnish with toppings of choice and enjoy.

Nutrition : Calories: 114; Protein: 5 g; Carbohydrates: 24g; Fiber: 4 g

9 781802 699876